C000099967

The Complete KETO Lunch Cookbook For Women

Healthy And Tasty Lunch Recipes For Weight Loss

Megan Kelly

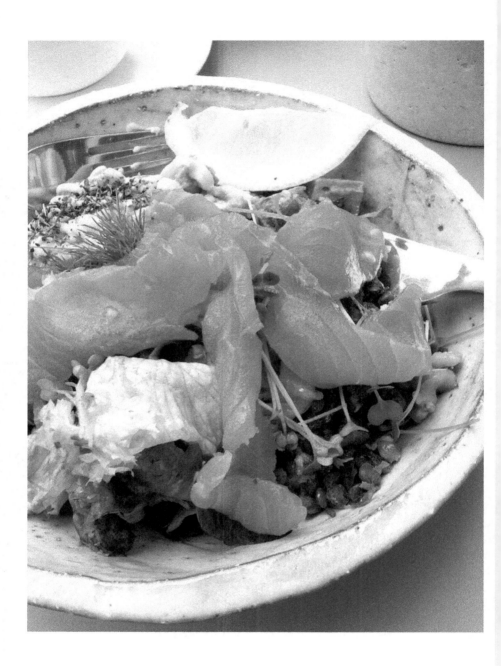

© **Copyright 2021 - All rights reserved.**

The content contained within this book may not be reproduced, duplicated or transmitted without direct written permission from the author or the publisher.
Under no circumstances will any blame or legal responsibility be held against the publisher, or author, for any damages, reparation, or monetary loss due to the information contained within this book. Either directly or indirectly.

Legal Notice:
This book is copyright protected. This book is only for personal use. You cannot amend, distribute, sell, use, quote or paraphrase any part, or the content within this book, without the consent of the author or publisher.

Disclaimer Notice:
Please note the information contained within this document is for educational and entertainment purposes only. All effort has been executed to present accurate, up to date, and reliable, complete information. No warranties of any kind are declared or implied. Readers acknowledge that the author is not engaging in the rendering of legal, financial, medical or professional advice. The content within this book has been derived from various sources. Please consult a licensed professional before attempting any techniques outlined in this book.
By reading this document, the reader agrees that under no circumstances is the author responsible for any losses, direct or indirect, which are incurred as a result of the use of information contained within this document, including, but not limited to, — errors, omissions, or inaccuracies.

Table of contents

Pizza Stuffed Chicken

Servings: 4

Time: 45 mins

Difficulty: Easy

Nutrients per serving: Calories: 402 kcal | Fat: 26g | Carbohydrates: 6g | Protein: 32g | Fiber: 1g

Ingredients

- ¼ cup Parmesan cheese
- ½ Tsp. Italian seasoning
- ½ Tsp. salt
- 1 cup pizza sauce
- 1 Tsp. garlic powder
- 1 Tsp. minced parsley
- 2 cups grated mozzarella, divided
- 2 Tsps. avocado oil
- 32 slices pepperoni
- 4 chicken breasts, about 6 ounces each

Method

1. Place the chicken breasts on a cutting board.
2. Drizzle oil on the chicken and season with garlic powder, salt and Italian seasoning.
3. In the chicken breast, position 1/4 cup of mozzarella. Over the cheese, add 4 slices of pepperoni.
4. In the prepared baking dish, put the chicken and drizzle it with the pizza sauce. Spread the sauce over the chicken tops to coat them.
5. Sprinkle the remaining mozzarella with it. Top with the slices of Parmesan and the remaining pepperoni.
6. Bake chicken for 30-35 minutes at 375°F.
7. Until serving, sprinkle it with fresh parsley.

Low Carb Chicken Patties

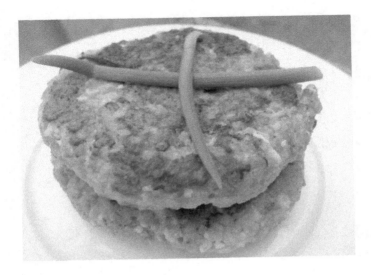

Servings: 10

Time: 16 mins

Difficulty: Easy

Nutrients per serving: Calories: 373 kcal | Fat: 25g | Carbohydrates: 5g | Protein: 33g | Fiber: 3g

Ingredients

- 2 cups cooked, shredded chicken breasts

- 2 Tbsps. mayonnaise
- 1 egg
- 2 green onions, minced
- 1 Tsp. fresh dill
- 1 Tsp. fresh parsley
- 1 Tsp. salt
- 2 Tbsps. butter, for frying
- 1/2 cup almond flour
- 1/2 Tsp. pepper

Method

1. To a mixing bowl, add all the ingredients except for the butter and whisk well to combine.
2. In order to scoop the mixture into your hand, use a medium cookie scoop.
3. Heat a large skillet with a heavy bottom over medium heat and add butter.
4. Add the chicken patties to the skillet once the butter has melted and cook until golden brown on each side, about 3 minutes on each side.
5. Immediately serve.

Ranch Grilled Chicken

Servings: 6

Time: 8 hrs 20 mins

Difficulty: Easy

Nutrients per serving: Calories: 494 kcal | Fat: 19g | Carbohydrates: 4g | Protein: 71g | Fiber: 1g

Ingredients

- ½ cup avocado oil
- ½ cup ranch dressing
- 1 Tbsp. apple cider vinegar
- 1 Tbsp. chopped parsley
- 1 Tsp. hot sauce
- 1 Tsp. salt
- 2 Tbsps. buttermilk
- 2 Tbsps. Worcestershire sauce
- 3 pounds boneless, skinless chicken breasts

Method

1. To a mixing bowl, add all but the chicken.
2. Add the chicken breasts and add the marinade to a baking dish or gallon zip top container. To coat the chicken, stir well.
3. For at least 30 minutes and up to 8 hours, marinate the chicken in the refrigerator. The longer you marinate the chicken, the more delicious it will be.
4. Heat the grill to a heat that is medium.
5. Remove the chicken from the marinade and let the chicken drip off a lot of it, then return it to the hot grill.
6. Grill on each side for 5-10 minutes until cooked through, depending on your chicken's thickness.

Lemon Caper Chicken

Servings: 4

Time: 25 mins

Difficulty: Easy

Nutrients per serving: Calories: 326 kcal | Fat: 19g | Carbohydrates: 2g | Protein: 36g | Fiber: 0g

Ingredients

- ¼ cup heavy cream
- 1 cup chicken broth
- 1 pound thin sliced chicken breasts
- 1 Tbsp. avocado oil
- 1 Tbsp. lemon juice
- 1 Tsp. pepper
- 1 Tsp. salt
- 2 Tbsps. butter
- 3 Tbsps. capers

Method

1. With salt and pepper, season the chicken on both sides.

2. Heat the avocado oil over medium heat in a big, heavy-bottomed skillet.

3. Cook the chicken, flipping for about 8 minutes halfway through cooking.

4. Remove the chicken and set it aside on a tray.

5. Apply the butter and the chicken broth to the skillet and bring it to a boil.

6. Reduce the chicken broth by half, about 5 minutes or so.

7. Apply the lemon juice and cream to the skillet and boil until the sauce is thick enough to cover the back of the spoon, stirring occasionally, for around 5 minutes.

8. Add the sauce to the capers and stir to combine.

9. Put the chicken back in the skillet and coat it with sauce. To re-warm the chicken, cook for 1 more minute.

10. Immediately serve.

Creamy Tuscan Shrimp

Servings: 4

Time: 17 mins

Difficulty: Easy

Nutrients per serving: Calories: 368 kcal | Fat: 29g | Carbohydrates: 8g | Protein: 20g | Fiber: 2g

Ingredients

- ½ cup sun-dried tomatoes
- 1 cup chopped spinach
- 1 cup heavy cream
- 1 Tsp. garlic powder
- 1 Tsp. paprika
- 1 Tsp. salt
- 16 ounces large raw shrimp, peeled, deveined, tail off
- 2 cloves garlic, minced
- 2 Tbsps. butter

Method

1. Over medium heat, heat a big, heavy-bottomed skillet. The butter is added to the skillet.

2. Attach the shrimp when the butter has melted and sprinkle with the ground garlic and paprika.

3. Cook for 5 minutes or until the shrimp is pink and opaque, stirring occasionally.

4. Remove the shrimp and set it aside on a tray.

5. To mix, add the sun-dried tomatoes, heavy cream, and garlic to the pan and stir well. Let the sauce cook over a low heat for 2 minutes to thicken.

6. Put in the spinach and stir thoroughly. Continue cooking over low heat for about 2 minutes until the spinach has wilted and the sauce has thickened.

7. Put the shrimp back in the skillet and coat it with the sauce. Sprinkle, to taste, with salt.

8. Immediately serve.

Low Carb Tamale Pie

Servings: 4

Time: 35 mins

Difficulty: Easy

Nutrients per serving: Calories: 580 kcal | Fat: 43g | Carbohydrates: 13g | Protein: 31g | Fiber: 5g

Ingredients

- ¼ Tsp. baking soda
- ⅓ cup heavy cream
- ½ cup coconut flour
- ½ Tsp. salt
- 1 cup grated cheddar cheese
- 1 Tbsp. taco seasoning
- 1/2 cup enchilada sauce, see note
- 2 cups shredded chicken breasts
- 2 Tbsps. 1:1 sugar substitute
- 3 large eggs
- 4 ounces diced green chiles

- 6 Tbsps. butter, melted
- Cilantro, hot sauce, sour cream, lime, avocado - for serving

Method

1. Preheat the furnace to 350 °F.
2. To a mixing bowl, add the milk, melted butter, and eggs and whisk to blend.
3. To mix, add the coconut flour, green chiles, salt, sugar replacer, and baking soda to the bowl and stir well.
4. In the prepared dish, spread the mixture and bake for 15 minutes. The cornbread in the center should only be put on top, but still quite jiggly.
5. To poke holes all over the cornbread, use a fork.
6. Drizzle the enchilada sauce on top of the cornbread.
7. Top a bowl with the cooked chicken and taco seasoning and stir to coat.
8. Over the top of the cornbread, arrange the chicken and sprinkle with grated cheddar.
9. Return for 10 minutes to the oven.
10. With your favorite toppings, serve.

Skillet Cabbage Lasagna

Servings: 6

Time: 35 mins

Difficulty: Easy

Nutrients per serving: Calories: 413 kcal | Fat: 29g | Carbohydrates: 14g | Protein: 30g | Fiber: 4g

Ingredients

For the lasagna:
- ½ onion, minced
- 1 clove garlic, minced
- 1 medium head cabbage, cored and chopped
- 1 pound ground beef
- 2 cups shredded mozzarella
- 24 ounce jar Rao's Marinara

For the ricotta topping:
- ¼ cup shredded Parmesan
- 1 clove garlic, minced
- 2 cups ricotta

19

- 2 Tbsps. freshly chopped parsley

Method

1. Over medium prepare, heat a large skillet and add the ground beef.
2. Brown the beef until cooked about halfway, breaking it up as it heats.
3. Apply the garlic and onion to the meat mixture and cook until the meat has cooked through, stirring regularly.
4. Apply and blend marinara to the meat.
5. Using the skillet to add the cabbage and gently stir to coat the meat sauce on cabbage.
6. Continue to cook over low heat for 15 minutes or until the cabbage is as soft as you like.
7. Remove the cover and replace the skillet with the mozzarella. To mix, stir well.
8. Add the parmesan, ricotta, parsley, and garlic to a small bowl to create the ricotta topping, and whisk to mix.
9. Spread the mixture of ricotta over the cabbage and cook for 2 minutes to warm up over low heat.
10. Immediately serve.

Cilantro Lime Shrimp

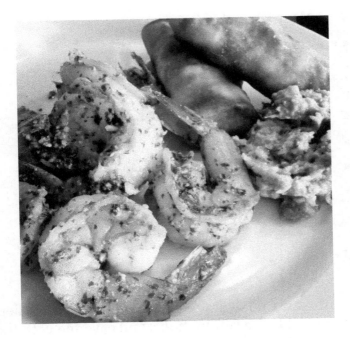

Servings: 4

Time: 11 mins

Difficulty: Easy

Nutrients per serving: Calories: 239 kcal | Fat: 7g | Carbohydrates: 2g | Protein: 38g

Ingredients

- 1 Tbsp. avocado oil
- 1 Tsp. salt
- 1/2 Tsp. cumin
- 1/4 cup chopped cilantro
- 1/4 Tsp. cayenne more to taste
- 2 Tbsps. lime juice
- 24 ounces large shrimp peeled and deveined
- 4 cloves garlic minced

Method

1. Heat the oil over medium heat in a large skillet. Sprinkle the cumin, flour, and cayenne with the added shrimp.
2. Cook for 4-5 minutes or until the shrimp is pink, stirring frequently.
3. In the skillet, add the garlic and cook for 1 minute more.
4. Remove and add the cilantro and lime juice from the sun. To mix, stir well.
5. Immediately serve.

Crockpot Cabbage Soup with Beef

Servings: 6

Time: 4 hrs 10 mins

Difficulty: Easy

Nutrients per serving: Calories: 205 kcal | Fat: 10g | Carbohydrates: 8g | Protein: 25g | Fiber: 3g

Ingredients

- ½ onion, chopped
- 1 carrot, chopped
- 1 medium head cabbage, chopped
- 1 pound lean ground beef
- 1 Tbsp. Italian seasoning
- 1 Tsp. salt
- 2 cloves garlic, minced
- 2 stalks celery, chopped
- 5 cups beef broth

Method

1. Brown the beef in a medium skillet over medium heat.
2. Add the onion to the beef and completely cook the meat.
3. Drain the oil and add onion and beef in a crockpot.
4. Top the crockpot and fill with the carrot, beef broth, Italian seasoning, celery, cabbage, garlic, and salt.
5. Cook for 4 hours on high heat.

Guacamole Chicken Melt

Servings: 4

Time: 22 mins

Difficulty: Easy

Nutrients per serving: Calories: 501 kcal | Fat: 30g | Carbohydrates:11g | Protein: 47g | Fiber: 5g

Ingredients

For the chicken:
- 1 Tbsp. avocado oil
- 1 Tsp. cumin
- 1 Tsp. garlic salt
- 1 Tsp. paprika
- 4 chicken breasts

For the avocado:
- 1 Tbsp. lime juice
- 1 Tsp. cumin
- 1 Tsp. salt
- 2 avocado

- 2 Tbsps. minced cilantro
- 2 Tbsps. minced red onion

For assembling:
- ½ cup grated Pepper jack cheese
- 4 slices bacon, fried crisp

Method

1. Add the oil to a large and heat over medium heat.
2. Season the chicken on all sides with paprika, cumin, garlic, and salt.
3. Add the chicken to the pan and cook until the chicken is fully cooked.
4. In a small bowl, add the red onion, avocado, cumin, salt, coriander, and lime juice and mash together with a fork.
5. Spoon the guacamole uniformly over each piece of chicken.
6. Break the pieces of bacon in half and lay 2 halves on each breast of chicken. Sprinkle cheese with it.
7. Cover the pan with a lid and let the cheese melt for 2 minutes.
8. Serve.

Creamy Tuscan Chicken

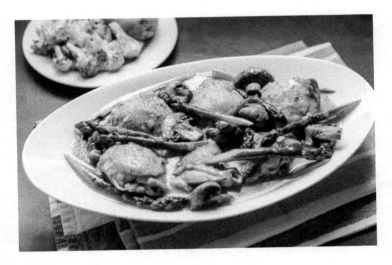

Servings: 4

Time: 20 mins

Difficulty: Easy

Nutrients per serving: Calories: 485 kcal | Fat: 32g | Carbohydrates: 8g | Protein: 42g | Fiber: 2g

Ingredients

- 4 thin sliced chicken breasts
- 1 Tsp. paprika

- 1 Tsp. garlic powder
- 1 Tsp. salt
- 2 Tbsps. butter
- 1 cup heavy cream
- ½ cup oil-packed sun-dried tomatoes
- 2 cloves garlic, minced
- 1 cup chopped spinach

Method

1. Combine the salt, paprika, and garlic powder and scatter evenly over the chicken.
2. Add butter to a heated skillet over medium heat.
3. Add the chicken breasts when the butter has melted and cook for 5 minutes on each side or until cooked through.
4. Remove the chicken and set it aside on a tray.
5. To mix, add the sun-dried tomatoes, heavy cream, and garlic to the pan and stir well. Let the sauce cook over a low heat for 2 minutes to thicken.
6. Attach the spinach and stir thoroughly. Continue cooking over low heat, about 3 minutes, until the spinach has wilted and the sauce has thickened.
7. Put the chicken back in the skillet and coat it with sauce.
8. Immediately serve.

Chicken Lazone

Servings: 4

Time: 20 mins

Difficulty: Easy

Nutrients per serving: Calories: 507 kcal | Fat: 37g | Carbohydrates: 3g | Protein: 39g | Fiber: 0g

Ingredients

- ½ Tsp. garlic powder
- ½ Tsp. onion powder
- ½ Tsp. paprika
- 1 cup heavy cream
- 1 Tsp. chili powder
- 1 Tsp. salt
- 4 Tbsps. butter, divided
- 4 thin sliced chicken breasts

Method

1. In a small cup, add the garlic powder, chili powder, onion powder, salt, and paprika and whisk to mix.

2. To season, sprinkle half the spice mixture on both sides of the chicken breasts.

3. Heat butter in a heated skillet over medium heat.

4. Add the chicken breasts and cook until they are cooked through.

5. Remove the chicken and set it aside on a tray.

6. Put the heavy cream and 2 tsps. Butter, and spices in the skillet. Whisk to blend well.

7. Bring to a boil and let the sauce get thick around 2 minutes.

8. Put the chicken back in the pan to coat it with the sauce.

9. Immediately serve.

Low Carb Zuppa Toscana

Servings: 8

Time: 40 mins

Difficulty: Easy

Nutrients per serving: Calories: 295 kcal | Fat: 18g | Carbohydrates: 10g | Protein: 20g | Fiber: 3g

Ingredients

- 1 cup heavy cream
- 1 pound spicy Italian sausage
- 1 yellow onion, diced
- 2 turnips, sliced, about 10 ounces total
- 3 cloves garlic, minced
- 4 cups chopped kale
- 4 slices bacon, diced
- 6 cups chicken broth
- Salt and pepper

Method

1. Over medium heat, heat a Dutch oven or big sauce pot. Add the Italian sausage to the pot and start browning the meat as it cooks, breaking it up.

2. Add the onion, bacon, and garlic when the meat is about half browned, and continue to cook and stir until the sausage is cooked completely.

3. Attach the turnips and broth of chicken and bring to a boil. Reduce the heat and cook for 10 minutes to simmer.

4. Add the kale and cook for 5 minutes or until both the kale and the turnips are tender.

5. Remove and stir in the cream from the sun. Taste and, as needed, add salt and pepper.

6. Immediately serve.

Low Carb Goulash

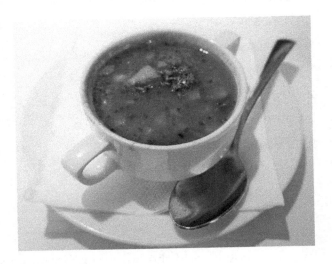

Servings: 8

Time: 45 mins

Difficulty: Easy

Nutrients per serving: Calories: 239 kcal | Fat: 16g | Carbohydrates: 7g | Protein: 18g | Fiber: 2g

Ingredients

- 1 bay leaf
- 1 cup beef broth

- 1 pound ground beef
- 1 Tbsp. Italian seasoning
- 1 Tbsp. soy sauce
- 1 Tsp. seasoned salt
- 1 yellow onion, diced
- 2 cloves garlic, minced
- 24 ounces Rao's Marinara
- 3 medium zucchini, chopped

Method

1. In a dutch oven, add the onion, garlic, and ground beef and brown over medium heat. Drain the fat and return the meat to the pan when the beef is cooked.
2. The remaining ingredients are added to the pot and brought to a boil. Simmer for 20 minutes, cover, and cook, stirring periodically, or until the zucchini is as soft as you like.
3. Prior to serving, remove the bay leaf.

Quick prawn, coconut & tomato curry

Servings: 4

Time: 30 mins

Difficulty: Easy

Nutrients per serving: Calories: 335 kcal | Fat: 26g | Carbohydrates: 7g | Protein: 19g | Fiber: 1g

Ingredients

- 1 green chilli, deseeded and sliced
- 1 medium onion, thinly sliced
- 1 tbsp tomato purée
- 2 garlic cloves, sliced
- 2 tbsp vegetable oil
- 200ml coconut cream
- 200ml vegetable stock
- 3 tbsp curry paste
- 350g raw prawn
- coriander sprigs and rice, to serve

Method

1. In a large frying pan, heat the oil. Fry the garlic, half the chilli and onions for at least 5 minutes.
2. Then, put curry paste and cook for additional 1 minute.
3. Add the creamy coconut, purée of tomatoes, and stock.
4. Add the prawns after 10 mins simmer on medium heat.
5. Cook for three minutes.
6. Sprinkle with the remaining sprigs of coriander and green chilies.
7. Serve with rice.

Peppered Mackerel & Pink Pickled Onion Salad

Servings: 6

Time: 15 mins

Difficulty: Easy

Nutrients per serving: Calories: 318 kcal | Fat: 25g | Carbohydrates: 7g | Protein: 13g | Fiber: 4g

Ingredients

- 100g bag honey-roasted mixed nuts
- 100g bag watercress
- 240g pack peppered smoked mackerel, torn into pieces
- 250g pack ready-cooked beetroot

For the dressing
- 1 small red onion , very thinly sliced
- 3 tbsp sherry vinegar
- 4 tbsp extra virgin olive oil
- pinch of sugar

Method

1. Mix the vinegar, onion, sugar, and some salt. Then, chop the nuts and dice the beetroot.
2. Divide the smoked mackerel and the watercress between six plates. Sprinkle nuts and beetroot over it and top with pickled onions.
3. Drizzle the dressing with oil in pickled vinegar.

Mediterranean Sardine Salad

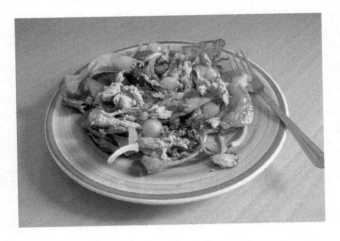

Servings: 4

Time: 15 mins

Difficulty: Easy

Nutrients per serving: Calories: 140 kcal | Fat: 10g | Carbohydrates: 1g | Protein: 10g | Fiber: 1g

Ingredients

- 1 tbsp caper, drained
- 1 tbsp olive oil

- 1 tbsp red wine vinegar
- 2 x 120g cans sardines in tomato sauce, drained and sauce reserved
- 90g bag salad leaves
- handful black olives, roughly chopped

Method

1. Divide the salad leaves, then drizzle over the capers and olives.
2. Cut the sardines roughly and put it into the salad.
3. Mix the tomato sauce with the vinegar and oil and sprinkle over the salad.

Smoked Trout, Watercress & Beetroot Salad

Servings: 4

Time: 10 mins

Difficulty: Easy

Nutrients per serving: Calories: 436 kcal | Fat: 38g | Carbohydrates: 7g | Protein: 17g | Fiber: 2g

Ingredients

- 1 tbsp creamed horseradish
- 1 tbsp French mustard
- 145g bag watercress, large stalks removed
- 150ml/¼ pint olive oil
- 250g pack cooked beetroot
- 2x 135g packs smoked trout fillets
- 50ml vinegar

Method

1. Put a bit of salt, ground pepper, olive oil, plus mustard, and vinegar in an empty bottle with a lid.
2. Refrigerate it.
3. Break the beetroot in quarters in a bowl.
4. Then, put 2 tbsps. of dressing and horseradish creamed and stir well.
5. Remove the skin and cut the tuna fish into pieces.
6. Mix the beetroot and watercress then put the smoked trout on top.

Avocado, Prawn & Fennel Cocktails

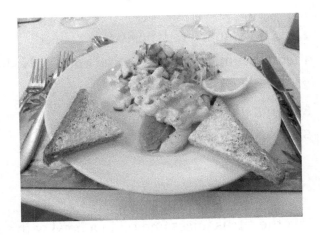

Servings: 4

Time: 10 mins

Difficulty: Easy

Nutrients per serving: Calories: 223 kcal | Fat: 18g | Carbohydrates: 2g | Protein: 13g | Fiber: 2g

Ingredients

For the dressing
- 1 segmented orange
- 4 tbsp extra-virgin olive oil

43

- juice 1 lemon

For the salad
- 1 avocado, quartered, peeled and sliced
- 1 fennel bulb, trimmed, halved and finely sliced
- 200g cooked king prawn
- 3 spring onions, sliced
- 55g bag wild rocket

Method

1. Mix the citrus juices and oil in a bowl with some pepper and salt to make dressing. Then set aside.
2. In a bowl, mix all the other ingredients, except the rocket, together with the half of the dressing and orange segments.
3. Put the rocket leaves into 4 Martini glasses.
4. Pile the salad, then sprinkle with the remaining dressing.
5. Serve

Spinach Artichoke Stuffed Peppers

Servings: 8

Time: 45 mins

Difficulty: Easy

Nutrients per serving: Calories: 178 kcal | Fat: 13g |
Carbohydrates: 7g | Protein: 9g | Fiber: 2g

Ingredients

- ¼ cup grated Parmesan
- ¼ Tsp. pepper
- ¼ Tsp. red pepper flakes
- ¼ Tsp. salt
- 1 clove garlic, minced
- 1 cup chopped baby spinach
- 1 cup cooked shredded chicken
- 1/3 cup grated Mozzarella
- 2 Tbsps. mayonnaise
- 4 bell peppers, any color
- 4 ounces artichoke hearts, diced

45

- 6 ounces cream cheese, room temperature

Method

1. Add water about 2 tbsps. in a bakery dish.
2. Cut pepper in half and place them in baking dish.
3. To a medium mixing bowl, add the spinach, mozzarella, artichoke hearts, red pepper flakes, cream cheese, mayonnaise, garlic, parmesan, salt and pepper. To mix, stir well.
4. To the mixture, add the chicken and whisk to blend.
5. Spoon the filling into each pepper evenly and put the peppers back in the dish.
6. Tightly cover the pan with foil and bake for 35 minutes.
7. Immediately serve.

Mozzarella Stuffed Meatballs

Servings: 4

Time: 25 mins

Difficulty: Easy

Nutrients per serving: Calories: 562 kcal | Fat: 37g | Carbohydrates: 7g | Protein: 48g | Fiber: 1g

Ingredients

- ½ Tsp. oregano
- 1 cup crushed pork rinds
- 1 cup marinara
- 1 large egg
- 1-pound ground beef, 90% lean
- 1 Tsp. garlic powder
- 1 Tsp. onion powder
- 2 Tbsps. chopped parsley
- 2 Tbsps. heavy cream
- 2 Tbsps. water
- 6 ounces mozzarella, cut into 12 small cubes

Method

1. In a medium mixing bowl, add the pork rinds, water, ground beef, onion powder, milk, egg, garlic powder, and oregano and blend well with clean hands to combine.
2. Divide 12 separate portions of the meatballs and form each piece into a tiny patty.
3. In the middle of each patty, put a slice of cheese and carefully fold the edges around the cheese to seal it in.
4. Be sure to seal the meatball completely around the cheese so that when baking it does not leak out.
5. In a 12-inch cast iron skillet that has been sprayed with non-stick spray, put the meatballs.
6. For 15 minutes, bake at 400°F.
7. Spoon marinara over each meatball.
8. Sprinkle just before serving with parsley.

Slow Cooker BBQ Chicken Wings

Servings: 8

Time: 1 hr 40 mins

Difficulty: Easy

Nutrients per serving: Calories: 495 kcal | Fat: 32g | Carbohydrates: 4g | Protein: 43g

Ingredients

- 1 Tsp. garlic powder
- 1 Tsp. pepper
- 1 Tsp. salt
- 1/2 cup chicken broth
- 1/4 cup reduced sugar ketchup
- 3 Tbsps. Italian salad dressing
- 4 pounds chicken wing pieces, thawed

Method

1. To a cooker, add the chicken wings.

2. Sprinkle garlic powder, pepper, and salt over the chicken.

3. Cook for 1.5 hour at a high temperature.

4. Take out the chicken and place on a baking sheet.

5. For 2-3 minutes, place the chicken on the broiler to allow the skin to become crisp.

6. Stir together the Italian salad dressing and ketchup in a small bowl until smooth.

7. Brush the mixture uniformly between the pieces of chicken.

8. Place the coated chicken to caramelize the sauce under the broiler and watch closely for about 2 minutes.

9. Take out of oven and quickly serve.

Lemon Baked Cod

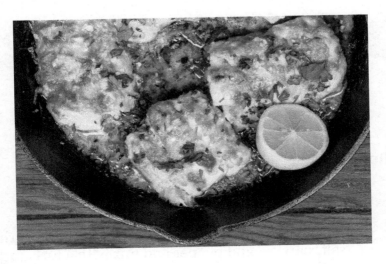

Servings: 4

Time: 25 mins

Difficulty: Easy

Nutrients per serving: Calories: 136 kcal | Fat: 12g | Carbohydrates: 1g | Protein: 7g | Fiber: 0g

Ingredients

- ¼ cup butter, softened
- ½ Tsp. pepper

- ½ Tsp. salt
- 1 Tbsp. lemon juice
- 1 Tbsp. minced parsley
- 1 Tsp. minced garlic
- 4 cod fillets, 4 ounces each
- 4 slices lemon

Method

1. Spray with non-stick spray on a baking sheet.
2. In a small bowl, add the lemon juice, butter, garlic, salt, parsley, and pepper and mix with a fork until well mixed.
3. Spread the butter mixture evenly and top with a slice of lemon over each cod filet.
4. Bake at 400°F for 15-20 minutes.

Teriyaki Chicken Stir Fry

Servings: 4

Time: 30 mins

Difficulty: Easy

Nutrients per serving: Calories: 271 kcal | Fat: 10g | Carbohydrates: 5g | Protein: 24g | Fiber: 4g

Ingredients

- 1 cup broccoli florets
- 1 cup cauliflower florets
- 1 pound boneless skinless chicken breasts
- 1 Tsp. chili paste
- 1 Tsp. minced garlic
- 1 Tsp. minced ginger
- 1/4 cup honey substitute
- 1/4 cup soy sauce
- 1/4 cup vinegar
- 2 cups chopped bell peppers
- 2 Tbsps. vegetable oil, divided

Method

1. Over medium-high heat, heat a large skillet.
2. Add vegetable oil about 1 tbsp. to a heated skillet.
3. Add diced chicken to a skillet.
4. Cook, stirring frequently, until cooked through.
5. Remove and set aside on a tray.
6. Add a different oil about 1 Tbsp. in the skillet.
7. Stir in the broccoli, cauliflower, and peppers and cook for 5 minutes or until tender-crisp with stirring frequently.
8. In a small cup, whisk together the vinegar, soy sauce, garlic, ginger, sugar, and chili paste.
9. Apply to the mixture and stir to coat. Cook for 3 minutes, stirring often.
10. Cook it while stirring for 2 minutes.
11. Immediately serve.

Broiled Lobster Tails

Servings: 2

Time: 10 mins

Difficulty: Easy

Nutrients per serving: Calories: 208 kcal | Fat: 10g | Carbohydrates: 5g | Protein: 23g | Fiber: 1g

Ingredients

- 2 Lobster tails
- celtic sea salt
- 1 tsp garlic powder
- 1 tsp smoked paprika
- 1 1/2 tbsp butter, divided
- 1/2 tsp white pepper

Method

1. Preheat the broiler to a high degree.

2. On a baking sheet or in an oven-safe bowl, put the lobster tails.

3. Cut the top of the lobster tail shell carefully down to the tip of the tail with sharp kitchen scissors or a knife, avoiding the meat. Devein and, if necessary, remove any grit.

4. Pull the shell down carefully, so the meat looks like it's lying open on top of the shell.

5. Slide a lemon wedge or two under the lobster meat, between the meat and the tail, to make it look even better.

6. In a small tub, combine the spices.

7. Sprinkle spices on them.

8. Using the lobster tail to add tiny pats of butter.

9. Place the upper middle rack in the oven.

10. Cook for about 8-10 minutes, until the meat is opaque and white.

11. Remove and serve with the drawn butter right away.

Rotisserie Prime Rib

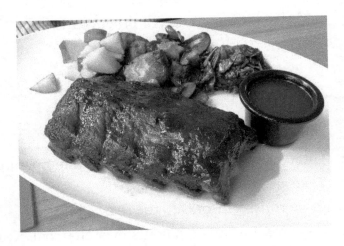

Servings: 2

Time: 4 hrs 45 mins

Difficulty: Easy

Nutrients per serving: Calories: 124 kcal | Fat: 8g | Carbohydrates: 6g | Protein: 8g | Fiber: 2g

Ingredients

- 2 prime rib roast, about 5 pounds
- 2 tbsp fresh cracked pepper

- 2 Tbsp. garlic powder
- 4 tbsp Italian seasonings or Aleppo pepper
- 4 Tbsps. kosher, Celtic, or other coarse salt

Method

1. Roast well.
2. Let it sit for around 2 hours at room temperature.
3. Take grill temperature to 350°F.
4. Place rotisserie forks in the roast.
5. Cook roast for 2 – 2.5 hours over charcoal. Keep the grill temperature about 350°F while cooking.
6. Remove the prime rib from the rotisserie and cover, loosely, with foil for 30-45 minutes before the meat rests.
7. Slice them and serve.

Smoked Brisket

Servings: 12

Time: 8 hrs 45 mins

Difficulty: Easy

Nutrients per serving: Calories: 137 kcal | Fat: 9g | Carbohydrates: 6g | Protein: 7g | Fiber: 1g

Ingredients

- 1 15 lb brisket

Brisket Baste:
- 1 cup beer
- 5 tbsp butter, melted
- 1/4 cup apple cider vinegar
- 1/4 cup beef stock

Brisket Rub:
- 1 tbsp brown sugar
- 2 tbsp chili powder
- 2 tbsp coarse ground black pepper

- 2 tbsp garlic powder
- 2 tbsp kosher salt
- 2 tbsp onion powder
- 2 tbsp paprika

Method

1. Start the Traeger grill.
2. Set the temperature to 225°F and preheat for 10 minutes with the lid closed.
3. In a small cup, blend the chili pepper, onion powder, kosher salt, garlic powder, paprika, and pepper together.
4. Season Brisket on all sides.
5. Place the brisket on the grill rack, fat side down.
6. Cook the brisket until the internal temperature exceeds 160°F.
7. Remove from the grill.
8. Double seal the aluminum foil with the meat and apply the beef broth to the foil package.
9. Grill, cook up to 204°F.
10. Remove from the grill once done.
11. Split and serve.

Smoked Turkey

Servings: 6

Time: 2 hrs 20 mins

Difficulty: Easy

Nutrients per serving: Calories: 110 kcal | Fat: 2g | Carbohydrates: 7g | Protein: 3g | Fiber: 2g

Ingredients

Brine:
- 1 cup kosher salt
- 1 gallon vegetable stock
- 2 Tbsp. black peppercorns
- 2 Tsps. savory
- 1 gallon iced cubes
- 1/2 cup light brown sugar
- 1 1/2 Tsps. allspice berries
- 1 1/2 Tsps. rosemary

Turkey:
- 1 turkey, 12-14lb

61

- Bag of charcoal
- Chips or chunks for smoking (fruit wood or oak)

Method

1. Bring all the ingredients to a boil.
2. Then, let it cool.
3. Put the cooled brine with ice in a cooler.
4. Put turkey in it and seal it in cooler.
5. Remove the turkey and air dry it to reach at room temperature.
6. Use a damp cloth or towel to cover the turkey.
7. When smoker reaches around 250°F add the turkey directly to the grates.
8. Keep rotating turkey and maintain fire at constant level.
9. Smoke the turkey for 30-40 minutes per pound at 235-250 °F before it reaches an internal temperature of 160 °F.
10. Smoke, cover, and let stand for 30 minutes prior to carving.

Brown Bag Herb Roasted Turkey

Servings: 8

Time: 3 hrs 5 mins

Difficulty: Easy

Nutrients per serving: Calories: 99 kcal | Fat: 9g | Carbohydrates: 4g | Protein: 2g | Fiber: 1g

Ingredients

- 1 carrot, chopped
- 1 celery stick, chopped
- 1 cup chicken broth
- 1 lemon, quartered
- 1 onion, peeled and cut into large pieces
- 1 turkey, 10 to 20 lbs, brought to room temperature
- 2 tbsp italian herb blend
- 6 tbsp butter, softened
- Large parchment paper bag, or brown paper shopping bag
- Salt and pepper

Method

1. To 375°F, preheat the oven.
2. Generally, rub the turkey with salt and pepper.
3. Within the turkey, place the celery, onion, lemon, and carrot as well as the collar and giblets.
4. Rub butter all over the turkey.
5. Sprinkle the herbs generously over the turkey.
6. Put the turkey in the bag and place it in a pan for roasting.
7. Within the turkey cavity, pour the chicken broth.
8. Fold the bag closed, and tuck it under the turkey so that it locks while it cooks in the steam.
9. Place the turkey in the preheated oven's center rack.
10. For the first 10 lbs, the cooking time is calculated to be around 2.5 hours, plus 12 minutes for each additional pound.
11. Remove from the oven and leave in the bag for 15 minutes until the turkey is completely cooked.
12. Then break open the bag, carve it, and serve.

Swiss Steaks

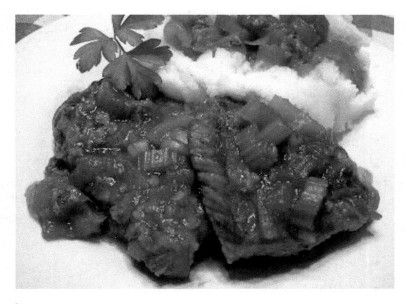

Servings: 4

Time: 3 hrs 10 mins

Difficulty: Easy

Nutrients per serving: Calories: 333 kcal | Fat: 19g |
Carbohydrates: 9g | Protein: 27g | Fiber: 3g

Ingredients

- 1 (14.5-ounce) can diced tomatoes
- 1 large onion, thinly sliced
- 1 Tbsp. Worcestershire sauce
- 1 tsp cracked pepper
- 1 tsp kosher salt
- 1 Tsp. dried oregano
- 1 Tsp. smoked paprika
- 1/2 can tomato sauce (7 oz)
- 14 oz beef stock
- 2 stalks celery, chopped
- 2 tbsp olive oil
- 4 cube steaks
- 5 cloves garlic, minced

Method

1. Preheat the furnace to 325 °F.
2. Generous steaks with salt and pepper.
3. Add olive oil to a wide pan or dutch oven and heat to a shimmery condition.
4. On both sides of the brown steaks, around 4 minutes per hand.

5. Remove from the pan when the steaks are browned, and set aside.

6. Add the onion and celery to the pan and cook until slightly browned and tender.

7. Stir in the garlic and cook until fragrant, about 45 seconds, with the onions and celery.

8. Combine onions, tomato sauce, spices, and sauce with Worcestershire.

9. Cook for about 5 minutes, before it bubbles.

10. Stir in the beef broth and placed the steaks back in the pan.

11. The cover pan has a close-fitting lid.

12. Braise for 2 1/2 hours in the oven until the steaks are tender and when pressed with a fork, the meat slightly pulls away.

13. Add up to 1 cup of water to continue cooking until the steaks are soft if the liquid cooks too much.

14. Place a little sauce in the pan and enjoy it!

One Pot Garlic Butter Chicken Thighs And Mushrooms

Servings: 6

Time: 25 mins

Difficulty: Easy

Nutrients per serving: Calories: 335 kcal | Fat: 24g | Carbohydrates: 7g | Protein: 25g | Fiber: 1g

Ingredients

- 1 cup chicken stock
- 1 pinch to 1 tsp red pepper flakes
- 1/2 cup diced cilantro, optional
- 1/4 cup parmesan cheese
- 2 tbsp lemon juice
- 4 chicken thighs, bones removed
- 4 tbsp butter, divided
- 6-10 cloves garlic, sliced in half or finely diced
- 8 oz cremini mushrooms, stems removed and wiped clean
- PINCH of salt

Method

1. Over a heated pan, add and melt the butter.
2. Then add chicken with a minute amount of salt.
3. Cook until chicken is turned to slight brown color.
4. Remove from pan and save left over oil.
5. Then, add garlic and stir.
6. Add mushrooms and to stop them from burning stir continuously.
7. Then, add butter second time and melt it.
8. Brown the mushroom and garlic without burning them.
9. Add cilantro and red pepper flakes.
10. Add lemon juice, stock, and cheese.
11. Boil and let it rest for 2 minutes to become thicken.
12. Add chicken thighs and let cook for about 8 minutes.
13. Take out of pan and serve!

Avocado Tomatillo Salsa

Servings: 16

Time: 15 mins

Difficulty: Easy

Nutrients per serving: Calories: 32 kcal | Fat: 2g | Carbohydrates: 3g | Protein: 1g | Fiber: 1g

Ingredients

- ½ cup of chicken broth or vegetable broth
- ½ Tsp. of salt
- 1 avocado, mashed
- 1 jalapeño, seeded
- 1 serrano, seeded
- 10 tomatillo tomatoes
- 3 garlic cloves, peeled
- 3 slices of white onion

Method

1. Begin by heating the oven to 425 °F.
2. Spray olive or avocado oil on a baking sheet lined with aluminum foil.
3. Cut tomato husks into four pieces after washing them.
4. Mix them with the whole serrano, jalapeño, and onion slices on baking sheet.
5. Sprinkle with a little salt and bake for about 10 minutes or until a nice char is created from the tomatoes.
6. To encourage them to bake evenly, flip the peppers and onion slices halfway through.
7. In a mixer, combine the tomatillos, peppers, garlic, onions, chicken broth avocado, and salt and mix until smooth.
8. Put salt to taste and immediately serve.

Oven Broiled Ribeye Steaks With Mushrooms

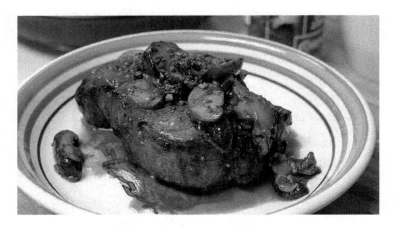

Servings: 4

Time: 55 mins

Difficulty: Easy

Nutrients per serving: Calories: 660 kcal | Fat: 60g | Carbohydrates: 7g | Protein: 13g | Fiber: 7g

Ingredients

- 1 tsp peanut oil
- 1/2 tsp celtic sea salt

- 1/4 tsp freshly cracked pepper
- 2 16 oz ribeye steaks
- 2 garlic cloves, crushed
- 3 tbsp garlic herb butter
- 3-4 thyme sprigs
- 8 oz cremini mushrooms, sliced

Method

1. Preheat an iron pan in oven.
2. Season the steak with pepper and salt, and let it stay at room temperature for 30 minutes.
3. Cut and slice mushrooms.
4. Add the steaks to the pan carefully, then the mushrooms, and shut the oven.
5. Flip the steaks after 4 minutes and stir up the mushrooms.
6. In a pan, add thyme and garlic.
7. Keep tossing and stirring steaks and mushrooms, depending on the thickness of steaks, until steaks are at your desired doneness.
8. Add butter on top of the steaks with pats of garlic.
9. Stir and leave to rest for at least 10 minutes before serving.

Grilled Spot Prawns With Garlic Herb Butter

Servings: 2

Time: 10 mins

Difficulty: Easy

Nutrients per serving: Calories: 660 kcal | Fat: 60g | Carbohydrates: 7g | Protein: 13g | Fiber: 7g

Ingredients

- 1 lb spot prawns
- 2 large cloves garlic, pressed or minced
- 2 Tbsp chopped flat leaf parsley
- 1 tsp fresh lemon juice
- Avocado oil
- 1/2 cup butter or ghee, melted
- 1/2 shallot, minced
- 1/2 tsp sea salt
- 1/4 tsp freshly ground black pepper
- 1/4 tsp red pepper flakes

Method

1. Prep butter for the spice. Melt butter over medium heat in a shallow casserole dish. Once it is warmed, add the garlic and minced shallot and cook until the butter is infused, stirring occasionally, for about 5 minutes.

2. Add the lemon juice, parsley, pepper, sea salt, and red pepper flakes and remove from the sun. Only set aside.

3. Prepare a spot of prawns.

4. Brush the flesh with some avocado oil on the foot. Set the prawn halves flesh side down on the grill when the grill is hot at 450°F.

5. For 90 seconds, barbecue.

6. Place the prawns carefully on a serving platter.

7. Serve with lemon wedges immediately and enjoy!

Spinach Strawberry Pecan Salad with Homemade Balsamic Dressing

Servings: 2

Time: 25 mins

Difficulty: Easy

Nutrients per serving: Calories: 524 kcal | Fat: 42g | Carbohydrates: 11.5g | Protein: 27g | Fiber: 4g

Ingredients

Salad

- 1 ounce crumbled feta cheese
- 1 ounce pecans (raw or toasted)
- 2 tbsp red onion, thinly sliced
- 3 oz strawberries, sliced
- 4 oz grilled chicken, sliced
- 6 oz baby spinach or spinach mix (170 g)

Vinaigrette Dressing (makes 1/2 cup)

- 1 pinch each salt and pepper
- 1 tbsp balsamic vinegar

- 1 tbsp red wine vinegar
- 1 tbsp water
- 1/2 tsp sweetener
- 1/4 cup light olive oil (or avocado oil)
- 1/8 tsp dried thyme
- 2 tsp minced red onion

Method

1. Make the dressing.
2. Slice the strawberries, chicken, and onions.
3. Put the ingredients in different bowls and drizzle over the dressing.

Cauliflower Broccoli Rice Salad

Servings: 4

Time: 18 mins

Difficulty: Easy

Nutrients per serving: Calories: 188 kcal | Fat: 18g | Carbohydrates: 6g | Protein: 2g | Fiber: 3g

Ingredients

- 1/2 cup walnut pieces, toasted (2 oz)
- 1/2 tsp black pepper (start with less)
- 1/3 cup avocado oil (or olive oil)
- 1/4 cup Champagne vinegar (or rice vinegar)
- 1/4 cup chopped parsley
- 1/4 tsp salt (or more to taste)
- 2 tbsp minced onion
- 8 oz broccoli florets
- 8 oz cauliflower florets

Method

1. Bake walnut pieces at 350°F for 15 minutes on a sheet or until they become fragrant.
2. Cool them with a tea towel. Rubbing the towel vigorously also removes walnuts bitter skin.
3. Take a small cup and add minced onions, vinegar and oil.
4. Pulse the cauliflower florets to rice grain shape and put in a serving bowl.
5. Similarly, pulse the broccoli florets, and mix both cauliflower and broccoli pulsed florets together.
6. Use cling film to cover the bowl for about 3 minutes and then microwave it.
7. Add ample oil in heated pan and add broccoli mixture. Cook it and stir for half a minute. Again, cook it for an additional 1 minutes. Now, let it cool under the sun.
8. Add walnuts and chopped parsley in riced broccoli mixture and blend them.
9. Add vinegar and oil according to your taste.
10. Immediately serve.

Big Mac Salad

Servings: 6

Time: 20 mins

Difficulty: Easy

Nutrients per serving: Calories: 368 kcal | Fat: 31g | Carbohydrates: 3g | Protein: 18g | Fiber: 1g

Ingredients

Salad

- 1 cup Tomatoes (chopped)
- 1 lb Ground beef
- 1 tsp Sea salt
- 1/2 cup Pickles (diced)
- 1/4 tsp Black pepper
- 3/4 cup Cheddar cheese (shredded)
- 8 oz Romaine lettuce (or iceberg if desired)

Dressing

- 1 1/2 tbsp Besti Powdered Erythritol
- 1 tsp White vinegar

- 1/2 cup Mayonnaise
- 1/2 tsp Smoked paprika
- 2 tbsp Pickles (diced)
- 2 tsp Mustard

Method

1. Cook beef over high heat in a skillet.
2. Season with black pepper and sea salt.
3. Fry while stirring and break beef pieces using spatula for about 7-10 minutes.
4. Make dressing. To do this, puree dressing's ingredient in a blender.
5. Refrigerate until ready to serve.
6. Mix the salad with beef and dressing.

Low Carb Jicama Pizza Fries

Servings: 2

Time: 25 mins

Difficulty: Easy

Nutrients per serving: Calories: 548 kcal | Fat: 48g | Carbohydrates: 17g | Protein: 17g | Fiber: 7g

Ingredients

- 1 package cut Jicama
- 1/2 package good-quality pepperoni
- 1/4 cup oil
- 1/4 cup shredded mozzarella cheese
- 3/4 cup Low Carb Pizza Sauce

Low Carb Pizza Sauce
- 3 medium cloves garlic minced
- 1 jar tomato sauce crushed tomatoes, no sugar added
- 1 tsp. powdered rosemary
- 1 tsp. dried thyme
- 2 tsp. dried parsley

- 1 tsp. smoked paprika
- salt to taste
- liquid stevia to taste (optional)
- 1/2 cup chopped yellow onion
- 1/3 cup + 1 tbsp. olive oil

Method

Pizza Sauce

1. Sauté the garlic and onions in 1 tbsp. of olive oil in a small skillet.
2. Mix every ingredient in a pot of medium size.
3. Cook for 3 minutes with stirring.
4. Cool and refrigerate it.

Pizza Fries

5. Toss the oil with the cut jicama.
6. Bake the jicama for 20 minutes at 400°F.
7. Remove from the oven, cover with pepperoni, cheese, sauce, and bake for another 10 minutes.

Low Carb Spinach, Strawberry, Bacon and Artichoke Heart Salad

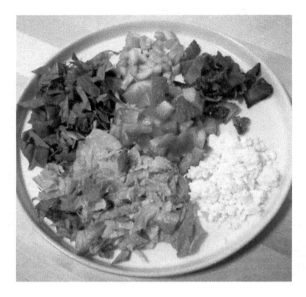

Servings: 4

Time: 15 mins

Difficulty: Easy

Nutrients per serving: Calories: 141 kcal | Fat: 10g | Carbohydrates: 4g | Protein: 9g | Fiber: 1g

Ingredients

- 3 oz. washed spinach leaves
- 1 tbsp. white balsamic vinegar
- 4 large fresh strawberries, sliced
- salt and pepper to taste
- 1/2 lb. bacon, cooked and broken into small pieces
- 1/4 (14.5 oz.) jar artichoke hearts + 1/2 the oil they are packed in

Method

1. Mix every ingredient in a bowl and serve.

Low Carb Chicken Tomato and Avocado Salad

Servings: 4

Time: 15 mins

Difficulty: Easy

Nutrients per serving: Calories: 341 kcal | Fat: 29g | Carbohydrates: 10g | Protein: 12g | Fiber: 5g

Ingredients

- 2 cups cooked, chopped chicken
- 2 medium avocados
- 1 tsp. garlic powder
- salt and pepper to taste
- 1/2 medium tomato, chopped (about 1 cup)
- 1/2 small yellow onion, chopped
- 2-3 large fresh basil leaves, minced
- 1/4 cup olive oil

Method

1. Mix every ingredient in a large bowl and use pepper and salt as seasoning to your taste.
2. Serve.

Low Carb Tuna Vegetable Salad

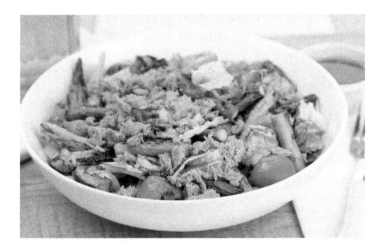

Servings: 2

Time: 10 mins

Difficulty: Easy

Nutrients per serving: Calories: 339 kcal | Fat: 28g |
Carbohydrates: 5g | Protein: 21g | Fiber: 1g

Ingredients

- 1 stalk celery
- 1/2 lime, juiced

- 1/2 medium cucumber, peeled
- 1/3 cup mayo, no sugar added
- 1/4 small red onion
- 2 cans water packed tuna
- salt & pepper to taste

Method

1. Mix all ingredients in a medium bowl and stir.
2. Eat as a single dish, or use salad as side dish.

Low Carb Keto Spinach Cobb Salad

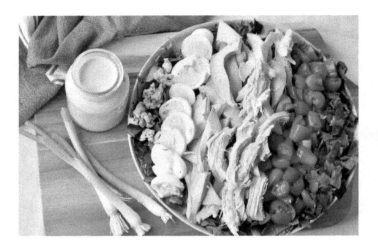

Servings: 2

Time: 10 mins

Difficulty: Easy

Nutrients per serving: Calories: 355 kcal | Fat: 23g |
Carbohydrates: 6g | Protein: 31g | Fiber: 4g

Ingredients

- 1/2 large avocado, cut into small chunks
- 1/3 cup chopped cucumber

- 1/3 cup chopped tomatoes
- 1/4 lb. good quality bacon, cooked and crumbled
- 2 cups raw baby spinach
- 2 large hard boiled eggs
- 4 oz. cooked chicken

Method

1. Put spinach in a bowl.
2. Add other ingredients on top of spinach and put dressing.

Avocado Tuna Salad

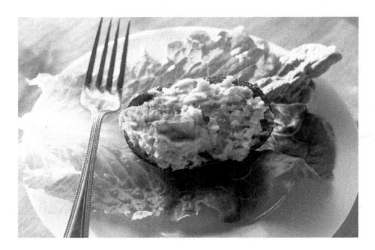

Servings: 4

Time: 15 mins

Difficulty: Easy

Nutrients per serving: Calories: 295 kcal | Fat: 29g | Carbohydrates: 9g | Protein: 2g | Fiber: 7g

Ingredients

- 2 Tbsps. yellow mustard
- 2 avocados, sliced and pitted

- 1/3 cup mayonnaise
- 1/4 Tsp. onion powder
- 1/4 cup celery, diced
- 1/4 Tsp. crushed red pepper flakes
- 1/8 Tsp. garlic powder
- 1 (6.4oz) canned tuna fish, drained

Method

1. In a small bowl mix mayonnaise, tuna fish, celery, onion powder, red pepper flakes, mustard, and garlic powder.
2. Put half cup of tuna salad in each avocado.
3. Serve.

Smoked Salmon Sushi with Cauliflower Rice

Servings: 24

Time: 25 mins

Difficulty: Easy

Nutrients per serving: Calories: 150 kcal | Fat: 10g | Carbohydrates: 7g | Protein: 8g | Fiber: 3g

Ingredients

- ½ avocado
- ½ Tbsp. "squeezable" ginger
- ½-1 Tbsp. soy sauce
- 1 small cucumber
- 1 Tbsp. rice wine vinegar
- 10 ounces frozen cauliflower
- 4 ounces smoked salmon
- 4 seaweed wrappers
- 4 Tbsps. cream cheese

Method

1. Heat the frozen cauliflower in a large skillet.
2. Add soy sauce, vinegar, and squeezable ginger. Stir well.
3. Add four chunks of the cream cheese.
4. Melt the cheese while stirring and make it is completely mixed with cauliflower.
5. Set aside the mixture and allow it to cool at room temperature. Divide in 4 equal servings.
6. Place four wrappers (seaweed) on a plastic wrap and spread cauliflower mixture on top of it.
7. Layer the cucumber strips, salmon and avocado slices with cauliflower rice.
8. Roll the wrapper to make sushi rolls.
9. Cut into half inch-thick rolls and drizzle dipping sauces and spicy mayo on them.
10. Serve.

Keto Ham And Cheese Rolls

Servings: 6

Time: 20 mins

Difficulty: Easy

Nutrients per serving: Calories: 198 kcal | Fat: 13g | Carbohydrates: 3g | Protein: 17g | Fiber: 0g

Ingredients

- 1 cup diced ham
- 2 eggs
- 1/2 cup shredded cheddar cheese.
- 1/2 cup grated parmesan cheese
- 3/4 cup shredded mozzarella cheese.

Method

1. Take oven to 375°F.
2. In a bowl, combine the egg and shredded cheese.
3. Mix well to blend them perfectly.

4. Add diced ham and stir well to blend.
5. Take a parchment lined or an oiled baking sheet.
6. Make round rolls by dividing the mixture in 6 equal parts.
7. Bake at 375 °F for around 20 minutes or when a faint brown crust is formed.
8. Serve.

Easy Keto Naan

Servings: 6

Time: 25 mins

Difficulty: Easy

Nutrients per serving: Calories: 411 kcal | Fat: 34g | Carbohydrates: 8g | Protein: 21g | Fiber: 4g

Ingredients

For the Naan:
- 1 1/2 cups Blanched almond flour.
- 1 tbsp Gluten-free baking powder.
- 2 large Eggs.
- 2 tbsp Full-fat Greek yogurt.
- 3 cups Mozzarella.

For The Garlic Butter Topping:
- 2 tbsp Butter.
- 1 tbsp Fresh parsley (chopped)
- 1/2 tsp Garlic powder.

Method

1. Take oven to 350°F temperature. Prepare a baking sheet with parchment paper.
2. Microwave sour cream and mozzarella in a large bowl, stirring every 30 seconds.
3. Add and mix the flour, eggs, and baking powder to the melted dough.
4. Knead until not sticky (add some almond flour to avoid stickiness).
5. Divide into 6 balls.
6. Spread the rolls on baking sheet.
7. Bake them until they are light brown in color.
8. Melt butter in pot and mix in garlic and powder parsley.
9. Bake naan in oven for 5 minutes after brushing garlic butter on them.
10. Then, Serve.

Pan Seared Scallops With Garlic And Lemon

Servings: 4

Time: 15 mins

Difficulty: Easy

Nutrients per serving: Calories: 190 kcal | Fat: 5g | Carbohydrates: 7g | Protein: 14g

Ingredients

- 1 lb scallops, defrosted, patted dry
- 1 tsp pepper, freshly cracked
- 1 tsp salt, celtic sea salt
- 1/2 cup white wine
- 1/2 lemon, sliced into half-wedges
- 2 tbsp garlic, diced
- 3 tbsp butter, grass-fed

Method

1. Melt the butter in pan.
2. Lightly season the dry scallops with pepper and salt.
3. Put scallops in a pan.
4. Heat until a golden crust is formed on one side of scallop.
5. Then, add garlic and let it brown but do not let it burn.
6. Add wine, lemon slices, and mix.
7. When scallops are browned and are springy, serve them topped with sauce.

Garlic Butter Broiled Lobster Tails

Servings: 2

Time: 15 mins

Difficulty: Easy

Nutrients per serving: Calories: 416 kcal | Fat: 31g | Carbohydrates: 12g | Protein: 24g | Fiber: 1g

Ingredients

- 1 tsp smoked paprika
- 1.2 tsp white pepper
- 1/4 cup minced garlic
- 2 Lobster tails
- 2 tbsp diced parsley
- 4 tbsp butter + 2 one Tbsp. pats of butter
- celtic sea salt
- juice of 1 lemon

Method

1. Add garlic and 4 tbsp butter in a large pan and cook on medium low heat.
2. Place lobster tails in an oven safe dish or on a baking sheet.
3. Carefully cut the lobster tail dodging the meat.
4. Pull the shell down and take out the meat.
5. Season with spices.
6. Add some butter.
7. Let cook in the oven for 10 minutes.
8. Add garlic and some butter to the lobster after 6 Minutes.
9. Remove and serve.

Low Carb Corn Dog Muffins

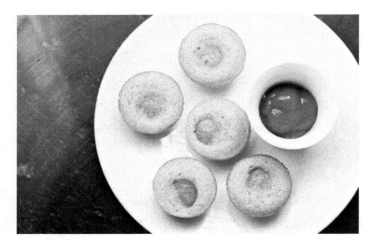

Servings: 4

Time: 35 mins

Difficulty: Easy

Nutrients per serving: Calories: 419 kcal | Fat: 24g | Carbohydrates: 8.5g | Protein: 42g | Fiber: 2.7g

Ingredients

- 1 pound boneless top sirloin steak, cut into 1/4-inch-thick slices

- 1 Tbsp. black and/or white sesame seeds
- 1 Tbsp. fish sauce
- 1 Tbsp. toasted sesame oil
- 1 Tbsp. unseasoned rice wine vinegar
- 1 Tsp. grated fresh ginger
- 12 cremini mushrooms, thinly sliced
- 2 cloves garlic, minced
- 4 (8-ounce) packages spaghetti-style shirataki noodles
- 4 green onions, sliced on a bias, white and green parts separated
- 4 soft-boiled eggs
- 5 cups beef stock
- 5 Tbsps. gluten-free soy sauce or coconut aminos, divided
- Pinch of red pepper flakes
- Sea salt and black pepper

Method

1. Use pepper and salt to season the steak
2. Rinse and soak the shirataki noodles.
3. Add the noodles to the heated pan and dry fry for 4 minutes.
4. Simmer the beef in a Dutch oven at medium heat.

5. Add the sesame oil, fish sauce, garlic, red pepper flakes, vinegar, ginger, and 4 Tbsps. of the soy sauce to the noodles.

6. Brown the noodles by frying for 5 minutes.

7. Add the sauce and noodles to the pot having the stock.

8. Scorch the steak for 2 minutes in the hot pan.

9. Add the green onions, the mushrooms, and the soy sauce to the skillet on medium heat. Fry them with stirring constantly.

10. Split the noodle among 4 bowls.

11. Top each bowl with the mushroom and mixture the steak.

12. Transfer the broth on each bowl.

13. Finish each bowl with sesame seeds, an egg, some green parts of green onions.

Keto Mongolian Beef

Servings: 4

Time: 35 mins

Difficulty: Easy

Nutrients per serving: Calories: 339 kcal | Fat: 19g | Carbohydrates: 1.9g | Protein: 37g

Ingredients

- ¼ Tsp. crushed red pepper flakes, optional
- ½ cup golden monk fruit sweetener
- 1 ½ pounds flank steak
- 1 ½ Tsps. glucomannan powder or xanthan gum
- 1 Tbsp. fish sauce
- 1 Tbsp. grated fresh ginger
- 1 Tbsps. avocado oil
- 2 Tbsps. gluten free soy sauce or coconut aminos
- 2 Tbsps. thinly sliced green onions
- 2 Tbsps. toasted sesame oil
- 3 cloves garlic, minced

Method

1. Cut the steak into thin strips, then into pieces. Set aside.
2. Mix the minced garlic, red pepper flakes, soy sauce, fish sauce, monk fruit sweetener, and sesame oil in a small bowl.
3. Add steak coated in marinade in a large bowl.
4. Refrigerate for 30 minutes to marinate properly.
5. Once the avocado oil is hot, add the marinade, steak, and grated ginger.
6. Cook the steak until color is brown.
7. Spoon out sauce and put in a bowl.
8. Use glucomannan powder to sprinkle on the sauce and mix the ingredients to thickens the sauce.
9. Serve beef with thick sauce and use green onions (sliced) to garnish.

Creamy Cajun Sausage And Potato Soup

Servings: 8

Time: 55 mins

Difficulty: Easy

Nutrients per serving: Calories: 323 kcal | Fat: 25.6g | Carbohydrates: 15.2g | Protein: 11.3g | Fiber: 1.8g

Ingredients

- ¼ Tsp. garlic powder
- ¼ Tsp. onion powder
- ¼ Tsp. rubbed sage
- ½ Tsp. dried oregano
- ½ Tsp. smoked paprika
- 1 medium carrot, diced
- 1 pound yukon gold potatoes, peeled and diced
- 1 red bell pepper, seeded and diced
- 1 small onion, diced
- 1 Tsp. sea salt
- 12 ounces andouille sausage links, sliced into rounds

- 2 cups full fat coconut milk
- 2 ribs celery, diced
- 2 Tbsps. olive oil
- 4 cups chicken stock
- 5 cloves garlic, minced
- pinch cayenne pepper
- pinch red pepper flakes
- sliced green onions, optional for garnish

Method

1. Heat the olive oil in a Dutch oven.
2. Then, add the andouille sausage and cook until color turns to brown.
3. Add the bell pepper, onion, garlic, carrot, and other seasonings to the sausage pan.
4. Sauté to tender the veggies.
5. Add the potatoes and chicken stock to the pot and boil them. Then, simmer for 20 minutes.
6. Stir in the coconut milk with andouille.
7. Simmer for 15 minutes.
8. Use green onions as garnish.

Lightning Source UK Ltd.
Milton Keynes UK
UKHW022030060521
383282UK00003B/338

9 781801 458818